# The Gems & Dementia, including Alzheimers:

A Guidebook for Care Partners

*Sponsored by*
*The Schriber Family Foundation*
*in memory of*
*Louis and Isabel Schriber*

Published by Cedar Village Retirement Community
5467 Cedar Village Drive
Mason, OH 45040
513.754.3100
www.cedarvillage.org

# The Gems & Dementia, including Alzheimers:

## A Guidebook for Care Partners

Seeing the unique and precious in the progression of dementia

Helping you to acknowledge and let go of what is missing while learning to celebrate and use what remains to make life well worth living until the end of the journey

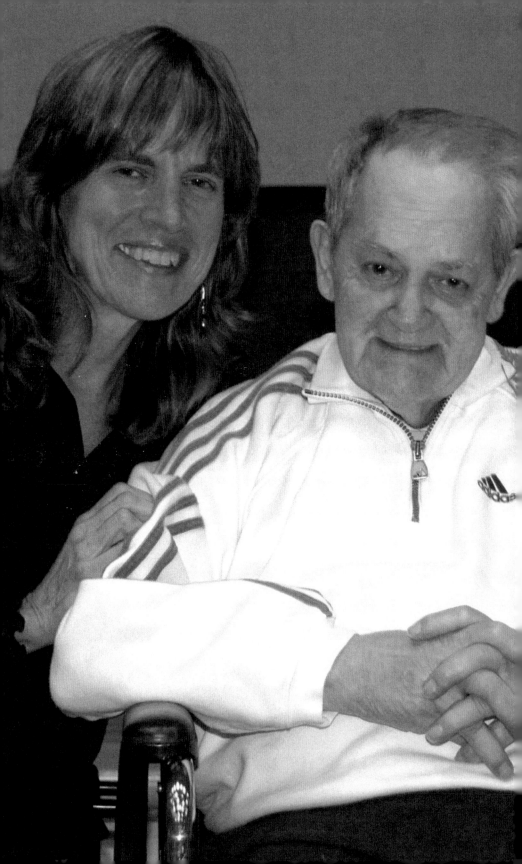

# Contents

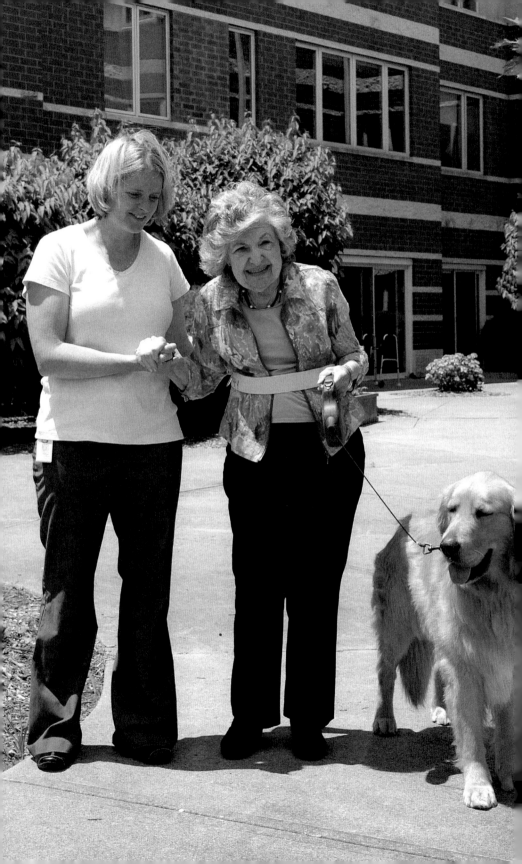

"We must not see any person as an abstraction. Instead, we must see in every person a universe with its own secrets, with its own treasures, with its own sources of anguish, and with some measure of triumph."

—ELIE WIESEL

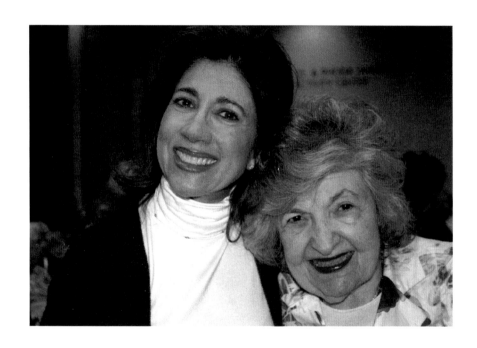

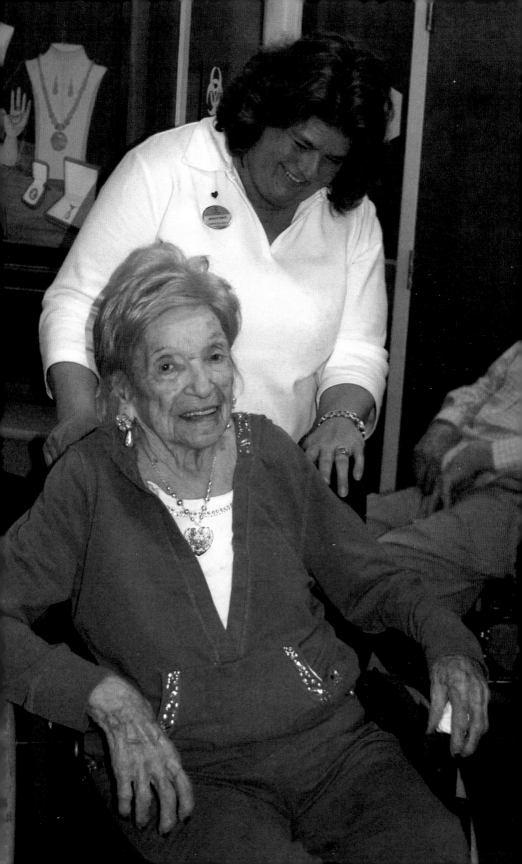

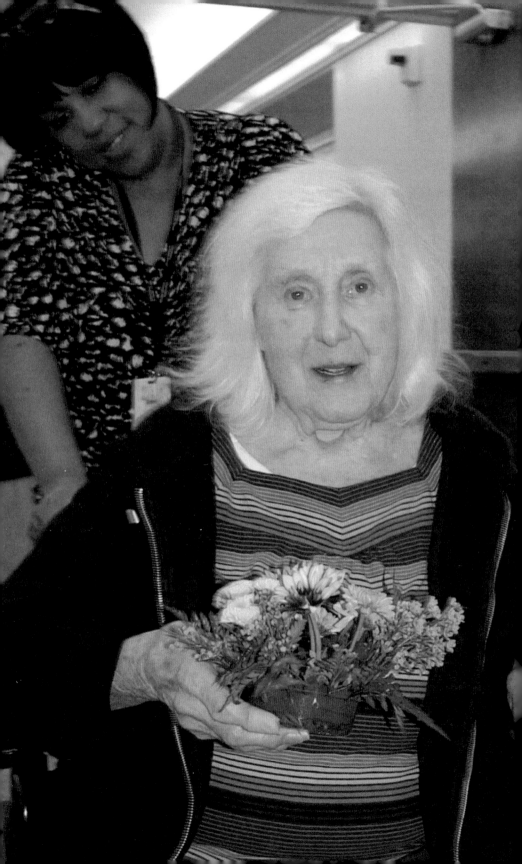

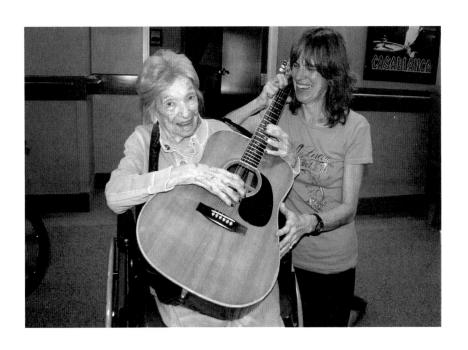

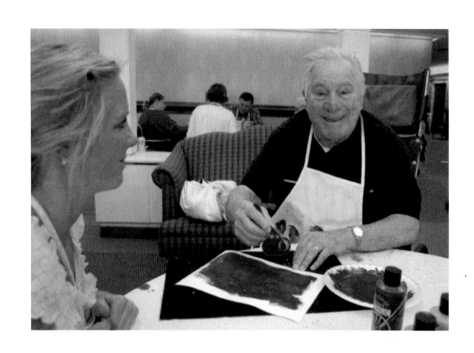

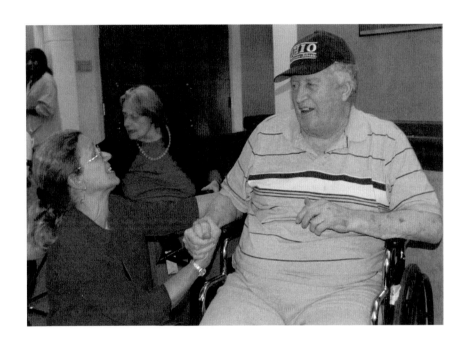

# How to Use this Guidebook

This booklet is designed to help family members, friends, and caregivers. Its purpose is to help everyone understand changes that come with advancing dementia or other impairments in thinking, reasoning, or processing information.

The goal is to provide better support and care when someone is living with this ever-changing condition, and to help them live fully in their moment! By appreciating what is changing and what is still possible, we can have interactions that are more positive, communication that is more productive, and care that is more effective and less challenging for all concerned.

The Gem Levels were developed after working with the existing systems of rating progression of dementia for over 20 years, and finding that they weren't quite enough.

- The first system was promoted and used by the Alzheimer's Association. It was a three point scale, 1, 2, 3–early, middle, and late. It is still helpful, as far as allowing us to get the general idea about where someone is in the disease process. Unfortunately, at this point in time, most people are diagnosed, not in the early stage, but in the middle stage. Since it is new information for families and caregivers, they are thinking early so their expectations are too high for where the person is functioning at that time. What they don't realize is that they may have been trying to cope with early stage issues for anywhere from one to five years, without knowing it.

- A second system was developed by Dr. Reisberg and is called the Global Deterioration Scale (GDS). It is a 7 point scale and goes from 1–7, with one being no cognitive decline and 7 being very severe cognitive decline (severe dementia). The emphasis is on what is being lost; what the person is no longer able to do and what performance abilities will deteriorate during that phase. It is accurate and it emphasizes that the pattern of loss most frequently copies the opposite of normal growth and development we see in infants, children, and adolescents. It works best if the person has a typical dementia like Alzheimer's disease, but not as well for Vascular, Lewy Body, or Frontal-Temporal dementias. These dementias have uneven progression patterns so the system is not as helpful.

- The third system was developed by an occupational therapist during her clinical work with people with a variety of cognitive issues. The system is based on her Cognitive Disability Theory and the levels are called Allen Cognitive Levels. There are six levels (6 to 1 –yes, the numbering is in the opposite direction of the other two systems). The huge plus is that it focuses more than just loss. It emphasizes what people would still be interested in, what they would be able to do, and what environmental support and care behaviors and cues would be helpful at the various levels. People can have a combination of levels present at once, and can move between levels throughout a day or task, depending on many factors and stressors and supports. I really liked this system, but there were two major problems with it. The numbering is in the opposite direction compared to the other two systems, meaning we would always be having disagreements in rating simply because of our association of numbers. The other issue is that numbers always have meaning. One is less than six and first is better than sixth.

So, I was looking for a system that would do some different things. I wanted a system with some way to:

1. Help us to see what remains and learn how to support and use those skills;

2. Provide consistent ways in which we can modify or structure the environment, the tasks, and our support for the best chance of success for each person in our care based on what they can do and what they need help to do;

3. Talk with each other in a way that did not carry so much baggage, so many values;

4. Develop a system that could be used by lay people as well as professionals;

5.  Talk about abilities in a way that is not hurtful or offensive to people who are living with the changes of dementia;

The Gem Level system is my effort to simplify a very complex process into a structured approach, for all involved, to better care for and support those living with changing abilities.

—*Teepa*

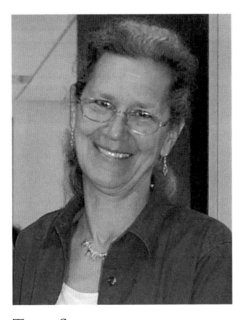

Teepa Snow, MS, OTR/L, FAOTA

# Key points to remember when using the Gem Level system:

1. Abilities are ever-changing. Use what you see, hear, and experience to help determine where the person is functioning in that moment or during a specific interaction to adjust your expectations, support, and behavior to match what is happening for them.

2. Gem Levels can and do vary during a day. As the person is faced with different settings, tasks, and people their ability to cope and respond may change regularly or unexpectedly. The existence and impact of other medical, emotional, and sensory conditions (vision, hearing, touch, balance, pain) can also affect Gem Levels. None of us perform the same when we are tired, stressed out, distracted, or in pain, as we do when we are rested, focused, and alert.

3. A person may show signs of different Gem Levels at one time. Use the support that seems to match the majority of the indicators as a first try. Notice how it is working, and modify as needed.

4. Gem Levels are not negative labels. They are indicators to guide us to help those we care for and care about. Any one of us can experience a Diamond moment. A good friend or partner will automatically move into a supportive mode for Diamonds and help us out,

not become frustrated or accuse us of being "stubborn, irritating, or stupid," and try to make us come back to Sapphire with arguments or anger.

5. If there is a sudden or unexpected change in Gem Levels, make sure someone who is monitoring the health and well-being of the person knows about it and is responding to this change. Sometimes the change indicates a next stage in dementia, sometimes it indicates environmental or emotional distress, but more commonly it may be an indicator of a physical problem, health issue, or condition that needs a good evaluation.

---

**On the next page**, there is a table that lays out the basics of each Gem–the jewel, the characteristics of the jewels, and the general behavioral characteristics of a person at that stage of dementia. Both remaining abilities and key missing pieces are noted.

Each of the following pages will explore the Gem in detail. For each one, the Gem will be described, remaining abilities will be high-lighted, lost skills will be noted, cues will be provided that match and provide better support and encouragement for the person at that level.

| Gem | Gem Characteristics | Cognitive Characteristics |
|---|---|---|
| **Sapphire**  | True Blue | Normal aging–no dementia–healthy and non-stressed. Brain mostly stays the same–slower, but still intact. Moments of feeling blue about changes/losses. Can do and learn new things–takes a lot of effort. It takes more time and more practice to learn. True to self–life-long patterns prevail unless there is an active decision to change. |
| **Diamond**  | Clear, faceted, sharp and cutting, reflects versus absorbs, high shine, expensive, zircon/diamond | Getting rigid–does best with the established routines and rituals. Can really do well at times–Can *shine*!–it seems planned or on purpose. Can be hurtful or say mean things without seeming to notice or care. Talks and worries a lot about cost, money, and expenses. Different people will see them differently. Can't seem to get it at times *or* won't let it go. Some family members not sure if it is dementia versus just being stubborn, mean, forgetful. |
| **Emerald**  | Green, on the *go,* going back in time *or* going somewhere to do something, flawed– making mistakes, vague– less clear in words, and deeds | Clearly no longer able to be independent. Making mistakes and not noticing or getting upset, but not being able to fix it. Will either want to be in charge *or* will look for someone to take over to guide and direct. Wants to be seen as an adult and competent. Language and comprehension more vague. Time and place traveling–going back. Needing meaningful engagement to fill the day–but may not know that. Getting lost in the sequence of events. Not picking up on internal cues–bathroom accidents, skipped meals or eating too often, missing baths, not changing clothing. |

| Gem | Gem Characteristics | Cognitive Characteristics |
|---|---|---|
| **Amber**  | Golden yellow, non-mineral, pine sap–item gets stuck on–more pine sap, each is unique focused on wants and needs, hyper-focused *or* not able to get focused, caught in a moment, *caution* light– no safety awareness | Living in a moment of time–not about the past. Focused on sensation–what does it look-sound-feel-smell-taste like. What can I do with items and space and sensations. Exploration without safety awareness. All about sensory needs and tolerance. Not aware of tasks as much–do I like it…or not? No ability to delay need or gratification. Harder to connect and spend time with me. |
| **Ruby**  | Red, hidden depths, skills are stopping, gets stuck moving or being still–can't easily switch, Takes more time to change gears, *slowing down* | Able to do big movements but not able to do fine detail skills (i.e., safe chewing, using fingers, using utensils well, safely moving around, more spills and slips and trips). Can grossly copy you, but not imitate–not understand what you want of them. Monocular vision only–losing depth perception. Limited ability to change gears–stuck either going or stopped. Needs gradual guidance to switch. Tends to repeat what went before, must guide to change. Losing fine skill in eyes, mouth, fingers, feet. Typically does better with rhythm–sing, hum, pray, rock, sway, dance. |
| **Pearl**  | Hidden in a shell, outside shell is ugly, layer-upon-layer, still and quiet, glows, shell closes reflexively with distress | Becoming immobile, curled into a fetal position. The person we know is locked away most of the time. Body is failing as the brain is failing, *but* the person will still have moments of connecting. Moments when the person reappears–layer by layer. Reflexes are overwhelming or missing. Connections must be made slowly and can't be maintained for long. We need to be able to let them go, not give up, but let go as they are leaving us. |

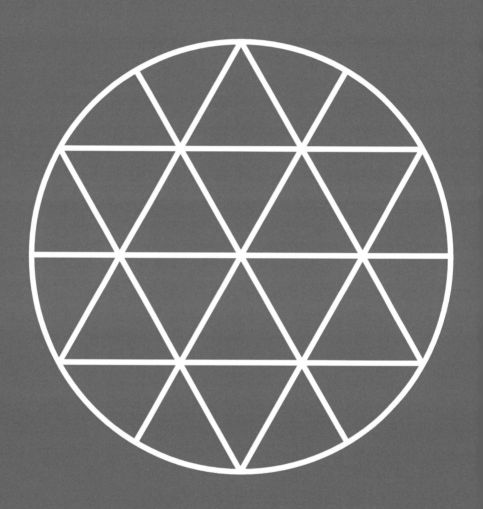

# Sapphire

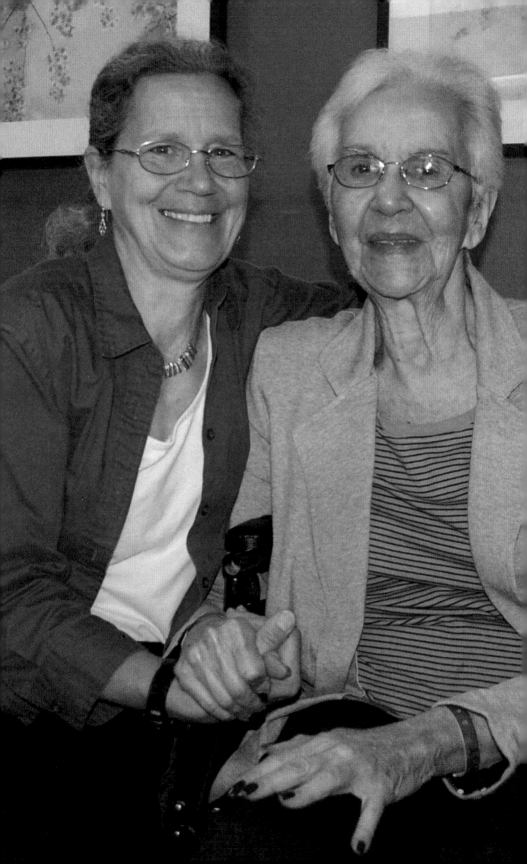

# Sapphire

## True Blue

### *Normal Aging, Not Dementia*

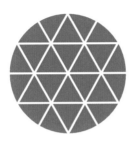

My brain is "true blue." There are changes, but they tend to happen to everyone and have been gradually occurring over time since my late twenties.

I am as I have always been, only a little more so. There may be moments or times if I am tired, stressed, sick, or frustrated that I can be diamond-like.

**Note:** If I am behaving like a Diamond, use those skills and approaches–but when I go back to baseline, I am fine.

Sometimes it is hard to find the words, but I can describe what I am talking about so you can get it. Word finding is harder if I am tired, ill, hurting, stressed, or trying to do too many things at one time. I may talk out loud as I am doing things or thinking it through–this is okay–I am giving myself cues and prompts. If I am fine with you filling in words, do it, if not be a little more patient and let me find the word myself, slow down a little.

Typically, I can still learn new things and change habits; however, it takes more effort and time to get it. Other health problems, sensory changes (vision problems, hearing changes, balance or coordination concerns), psychological or mental health concerns (depression, anxiety, personality disorders, etc.), medication effects or side effects, or chronic pain issues may affect abilities and behavior but cognitive abilities are pretty much intact.

I will be able to remember important commitments and pieces of information, but I may need to use reminders and prompts. I will typically need to use aids for details and complex instructions or information. I will have to practice more to get things and may get frustrated if you try to go too fast, go over it only once or twice, or point out that I am not as fast or sharp as I used to be.

Seeking out my preferences and honoring my choices is important whenever possible. If there is something you really want or need me to do, you will want to consider who I am and how I like to get information, process information, and make decisions before you bring it up.

**Note:** If I have never been like this, maybe I have always been a Diamond. Try using the Diamond skills to help and cope. It should help both of you!

## *Helpful Tips for Sapphires* |

1. I will usually want more time to make choices or decisions–give the information and then let me think about it before you need an answer.

2. I will typically resent takeover unless I ask or want you to do so, based on my health or your skill or knowledge.

3. I can use logic and reason at the same level as I have for most of my life, so use what you know about me to help determine how, when, who, what types of questions to ask, information to share, and support to offer.

4. If I have preferred learning styles or I tend to like specific prompts (notes, calendars, calls, reminders, alarms) try to use that mode. For example: to do lists, grocery lists, daily or weekly pill boxes, cell phone or watch alarms, white board notes, handouts, written or picture instruction sheets, CD (audio) or DVD (video) demonstrations and prompts, written contracts or agreements.

5. Due to common hearing issues, make sure only one person talks at a time when important information is being discussed. Allow time for questions and always ask me to share what I was told (this allows you to make sure I heard and understood what you thought you shared). It also allows me to rehearse the information once, and provides an opportunity to address any missed items, misheard information, or misunderstood concepts.

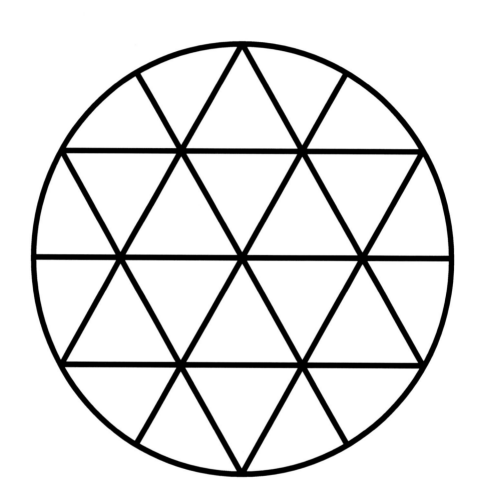

# Diamond

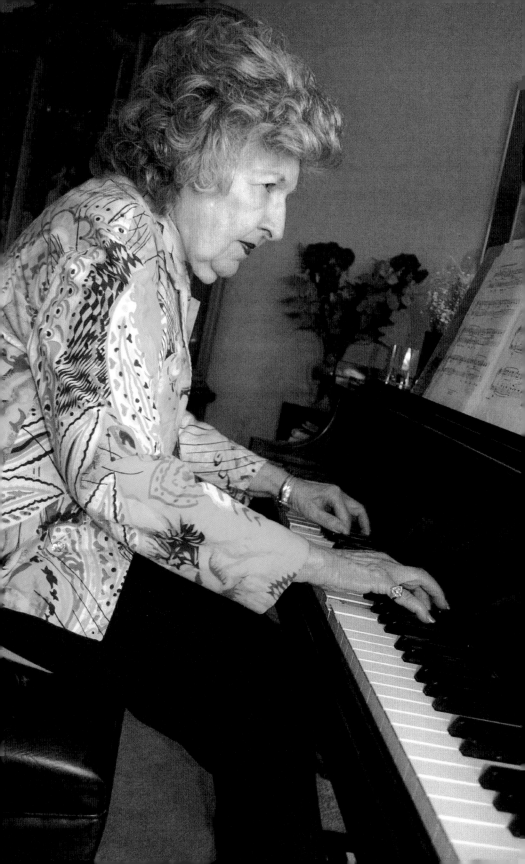

# Diamond

## Clear, Sharp, Rigid, Reflective

### First Signs of Change or Signals of a Stressed Brain

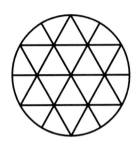

My brain is still clear and sharp, I can and do shine at times, at other times I can be cutting or hard, which may not be typical for me at all. I have many facets, so everyone sees me differently (potentially causing conflict among my care team and/or family members). I tend to reflect your concerns back, they are bounced around inside and I work to hide them, or I mention them and we all treat them as just normal getting old things … when they happen more frequently, are more intense, or are not me, it might not be.

It is usually hard to tell if I am just being difficult or stubborn or if I am having changes in my abilities.

You may notice that I am getting very rigid and inflexible in how I like things, do things, and want things or that I seem less and less aware of boundaries or limits in my expectations. I seem to think I am the center of what is going on and I want to be special and unique, not seeming to care about others.

I struggle a lot with changes and new routines, expectations, settings, or situations. I may or may not be aware of these changes. I am becoming accusatory– thinking others are trying to trick me or conspire against me. I am also very focused on money, finances, expenses, making statements like "As much as this costs…" or "I never thought you would be more interested in the money than your own…"

I will want to keep roles, habits, environments, 'rules' and supports just like they have 'always been', even though they may not be working.

I do tend to retain respect for authority figures and I know who authority figures are (doctor, administrator, lawyer, nurse, rabbi, oldest child, policeman…)

I may become very angry or anxious or sad if you try to get me to understand that I am not doing as well as I used to; that I am not being "logical," that I am not "following the rules," or that I am being "mean."

It is very possible that people who do not know me well will not notice the changes at first. It is also possible because I am good at social chit-chat and have good cover skills that brief visits and social settings will not allow the other people in my life to see how much I am struggling or losing some of my higher quality skills in language, problem solving, way-finding, detail organizing, and new information retention.

It is also possible that if you are around me all the time, you may not notice how much I am changing, because you get used to it. You don't notice how often you are filling n missing words, reminding me about appointments, or getting me where I need to be.

It is also possible if you only see me occasionally, you may not notice. My brain will notice you as something special and will produce more chemicals and make me seem better than I usually am (this happens at the doctors, driving tests, and public events. This makes it seems like I am just not trying other times, which is not the case…it's all about chemistry.)

You may notice that I ask the same questions about recent information over and over and also tell old stories or repeatedly relate emotionally charged stories. So you may find yourself saying, "Remember I told you…" or "Don't you remember?" Or when I say, "Did I ever tell you…?" You may think or say, "Only about 20 times!" This happens because you get tired of hearing it or frustrated with my repetition, but for me it is new information each time.

I am also struggling with words at times. I talk my way around them, or use vague words at times. Usually nouns are the first words to be missing. So I might say, "Where is my…you know the thing I use to pay the bills…?" (when I am looking for my checkbook).

I am also beginning to have some trouble with understanding complex phrases and difficulty in keeping up with changes in topics. My speech may seem a little off-target or tangential.

## Helpful Tips for Diamonds |

1. Recognize the changes and be willing to modify your

approach and expectations when the symptoms are active–when I am a Diamond–you change!

2. Stop arguing! Give up reality orientation! Stop needing to be right! Learn how to help and support without being bossy or taking over completely.

3. Be willing to say you are sorry. "I'm sorry, I was trying to help," "I'm sorry I made you angry/sad/frustrated/anxious/feel stupid," "I'm sorry this happened," or "I'm sorry, this is hard!"

4. When I ask or tell you repeatedly about something– get rid of the words "Remember" and "Don't you remember?" instead use this sequence:

   • Repeat the gist of what I just said.
   • Offer the information I asked about (using a combination of visual and verbal prompts).
   • Keep your voice and manner calm and friendly.
   • If you are getting tired or frustrated–take a break, get help, or after you respond, try getting me onto another subject or topic by asking for my help, providing something different and interesting to do, or use humor rather than negative emotions to cope.

5. Limit sharing of advance information, appointments, vacations, or plans if it creates distress and anxiety.

6. Listen to my old stories and learn the details of them

(you will need to know them as the disease progresses)–When I ask, "Did I ever tell you about…?" instead of saying "yes" or "no," use a few of the words and then state, "Tell me about it!" with enthusiasm and interest. Keep in mind that I am trying to talk with you, *but* I want to be in charge of the conversation. I don't remember that I already told you, *but* I do want to connect with you.

7. Let me keep as many old routines and habits as possible, but if they aren't working indicate that an authority figure says we have to do something different at least for now…we need to *try* this…it's a rule for everyone. You need me to help you out, not because of me, but because of you or someone else. In other words, it's not about me being incompetent or unable, but about others.

8. Help me establish and maintain a healthy rhythm to my day–balanced among productive, wellness, restorative, and leisure activities. Use environmental and social support to foster this lifestyle and rhythm. Sustain engagement or work to gradually improve the balance–baby steps!

9. Investigate my safety in independent living skills–driving or public transportation use, financial management, care of another, medication and health condition management, meals and food management, home and car maintenance.

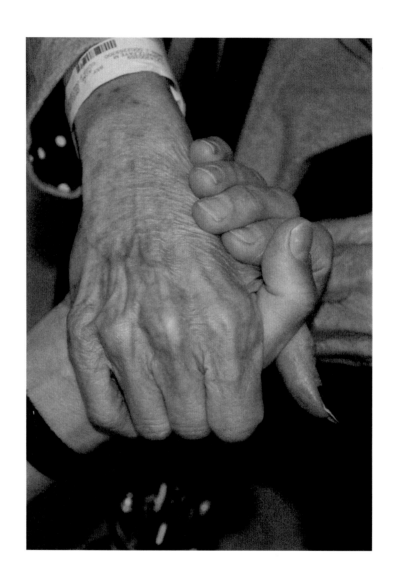

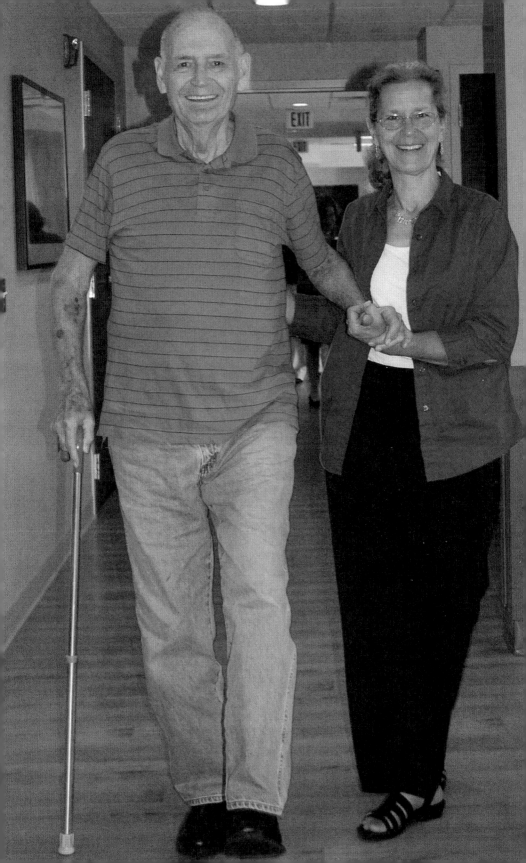

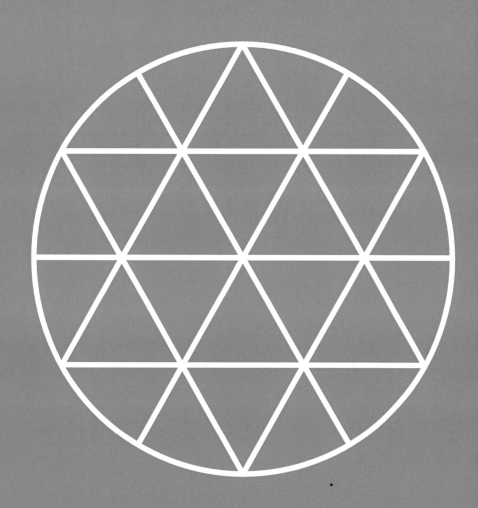

# Emerald

.

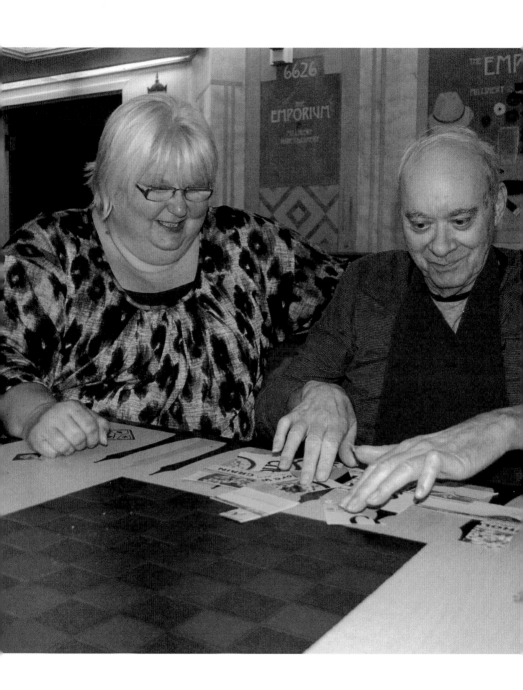

# Emerald

## Green, Vague, Flawed Internally

### *Moderate Symptoms of Cognitive Changes*

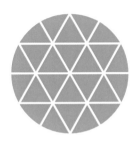

The changes I am experiencing are now much more visible to others, *but* I have limited or no awareness of my flaws and my loss of abilities. I make mistakes. I am on the go–sometimes I am going back in time, and sometimes I am going somewhere but not clear about where or when. I want to do things, supervise you doing things, or watch you, but I struggle to get it right. My changes and losses get more apparent as the day grows late: shorter cycles on repeats, more emotionally fragile, needing more cues to get it. I am just not as clear or sharp.

I pay more attention to what I see than what I hear. If I see it I do it, if I don't see it, I miss it–skip care routines and think I have already done them or say I will do them later (but don't) or do them over and over in a single day.

My functional vision is mostly binocular–limited for peripheral awareness around the edge of my visual field–I lose awareness of what is to the sides, low, and high. I may start walking while looking down more, miss what is a surface right in front of me (my food or drink, my glasses, the dog) but focus on something interesting across the room, ignoring what is closer.

I may think I am in a different time and place in my life, especially later in the day or when I am stressed or not feeling well, or in an unfamiliar place or even in a familiar one. This means I may not recognize you for who you are t me in this time period. I may think my children are small, not grown-up, so I can't see you as my daughter and may think you are a nice lady I know or a friend, or my mother. I may not know the person I have been married to for 50 years because I am looking for the man in the wedding picture. I may think I am very young and look for my hom from then or my family from then. I may insist that I need to go home, even though I am home. I may think strangers are friends and friends are strangers in these moments. I hurt you, I am sorry, but I am lost in my life and can't com back as you want me to.

Although I can chit-chat, I am struggling to get words out–losing nouns, misspeaking at times, describing words versus saying the word, or using visual cues rather than saying what I want to say.

I am making mistakes in some of my personal care, but I will not want you to help me if it makes me feel incompetent or stupid. I will resent being treated like a child if you just try to physically assist or help.

My emotions may get out of control easily and I may go over the top–usually it is worse in the later afternoon or evening because I am wearing out. I can really enjoy events, but there may be a payback later due to chemical drain and old memories taking over–like time travel.

I get very concrete in my language comprehension and am missing a quarter of the words in a sentence. When you try to explain something or reason with me, I will get lost or upset because I can't hold onto it or get it and I can tell you are not happy about it (tone of voice and facial expression).

I don't know how to organize or use my free time anymore and may continually seek out guidance. "What do I do now? ...Where should I go?" or I may just stay in my cave, a familiar location, but not really do much.

My brain will fill in the blank spots with false memories (confabulation) which makes it seem like I am making things up or lying–I am not–my brain is lying to me–if you try to argue with me about it or get me to get it I will tend to become more suspicious, resentful, and fearful–this makes care harder to deliver.

I generally can remember my feelings toward you or others when they are strong, but I won't remember the details of why I feel that way, so my brain will make up information so it makes sense to me–I can't be logical or rational about this.

I will either think I am more competent and able than I am, or seek out constant guidance reassurance and help. Both extremes will wear on you. Constant reassurance will wear you out, as I can't hold on to what you say or what we just did. Overestimation of skills and abilities results in changes in the quality of my personal care routines and my appearance. It can also result in problems with personal hygiene, a total lack of care routines, unsafe task performance, and major problems in managing other health conditions.

## *Helpful Tips for Emeralds* | ✦

1. Learn the importance of "So what?"–before deciding to do something about an error, a difference, or something that is not how I have always been–stop and decide…Is it worth it? Do you really need to do something about this–right now? Will it matter in five minutes, five days, five months, or five years?

2. Greet before you treat!–Learn the importance of getting connected to me (establishing the relationship) each time before you try to address or fix something you noticed that I did wrong or is "flawed."

3. Learn how to do things with me, not to me or for me– let me be a partner and feel that we are in this together.

4. If I am lost in my life, accept that in this moment I am lost and I need you to stay calm, get connected in a way I can understand it, listen to me and try to figure out what I need and meet that need. So, instead of trying to get me to understand the reality–
   a. Offer your name in greeting, not the relationship– you may need to use my name not our relationship ("Hi Mary, it's John." –not "Hi Mom, it's me.")

b. If I don't seem to know who you are to me, Let it go—relax and be a friend not a family member.

c. If I say, "I want to go home," or that I am "looking for my mother," don't use reality orientation or argue—instead:

    i. Get connected using PPA. (see page 64)

    ii. Repeat my words—"You need to get home…" "You are feeling a need for your mother…"

    iii. Then make an emotionally supportive comment, "You have always loved being at home…" or "Sounds like you are really missing your mother…," pause and listen to what I say…

    iv. If language is not too much of a problem, offer, "Tell me about your…home or mother."

    v. If language is a problem, offer information about the place or person, "You have something you need to do at home…?" "Is your mother a great cook?…Do you like her dinners or desserts better?" Not distraction but redirection.

    vi. Consider taking the person to a more unfamiliar place for a short period (on a walk or ride) then bring them back and they may reconnect with the place and be okay.

5. When you want me to do something, use visual cues first. Show me—point, gesture, use props, demonstrate, do it along-side me, not to me.

6. Think before you speak.
    a. Limit how much you say. Pause after a sentence. Slow it down a little and wait for my responses.
    b. Make sure your visual cues match your verbal information (show then tell).
    c. When you change subjects or topics, give a stronger cue of a switch–visual and verbal "Oh…"
    d. Notice things out loud and with gestures…"Isn't that interesting…"
    e. Offer either/or choices, "Would you like something hot or cold to drink?" not, "What do you want to drink?"
    f. If I say, "I need something," say, "You need something?" pause, then add, "Tell me more about it," or "Could you show me what you'd do with it?" Don't ask me what I need. I either don't know or won't be able to find the word…that is why I used "something."

7. Build a daily routine and schedule–that provides structure and sequence that is regular–be careful about special events and surprises–keep them small, short, and be willing to let it go if it is not working for me.

8. If what you want is not working, stop and back off, change something and then re-approach and try again.

9. You will need to learn how to respond, not react to what I do or say–it may feel like work at times.

0.  Use humor, laugh with me not at me–If I don't find it funny, stop and apologize.

1.  Break tasks, activities, and expectations down into smaller steps, less at a time. Help me want to get up and get going, before you talk about getting personal care done or what will happen later. Try to think about what I would like to do, not what needs to be done.

2.  Ask if I can help you, not that you need or want to help me. Let me feel like I still matter and make a difference. Share tasks with me, don't do for me or try to do to me.

3.  Consider writing out and sharing a first person narrative of my life story with key pieces of information with others involved in my care, so they can help better, by knowing who and how I have been.

4.  If you are aware, share information about whether I typically like to physically do things and stay busy/active, socially engage, or just observe others and activity. This will help team members know how to help build a day that works well for me.

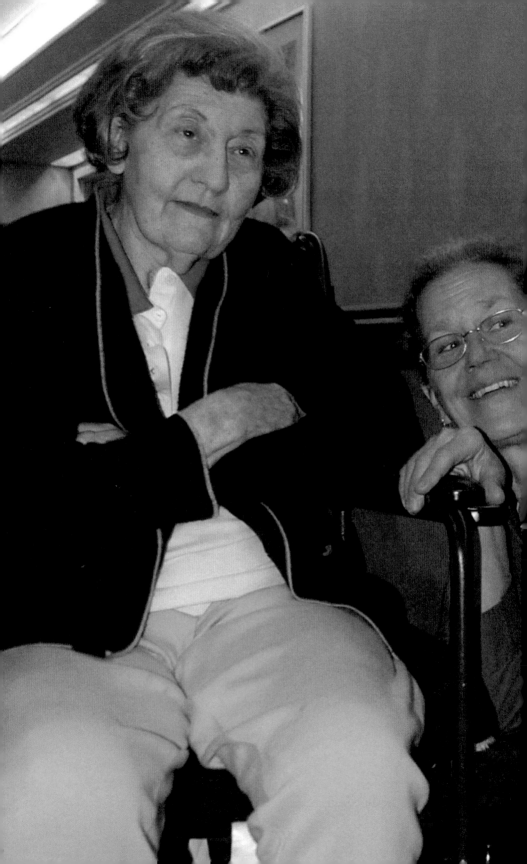

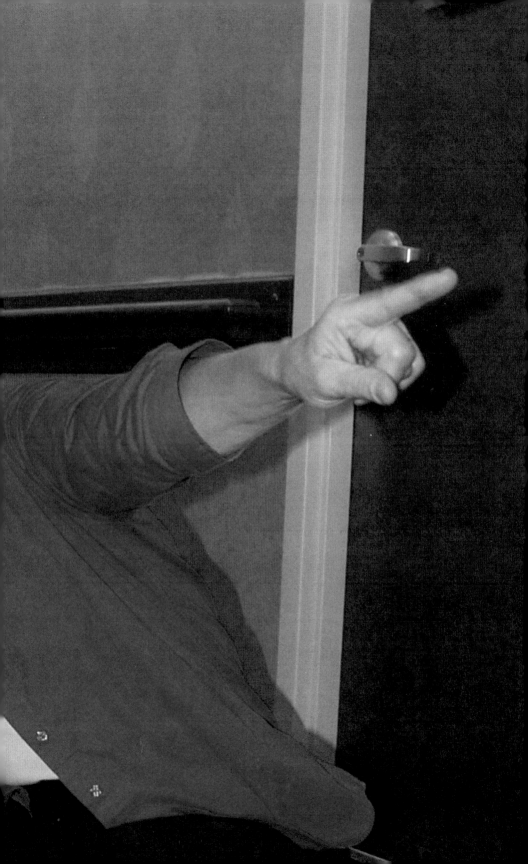

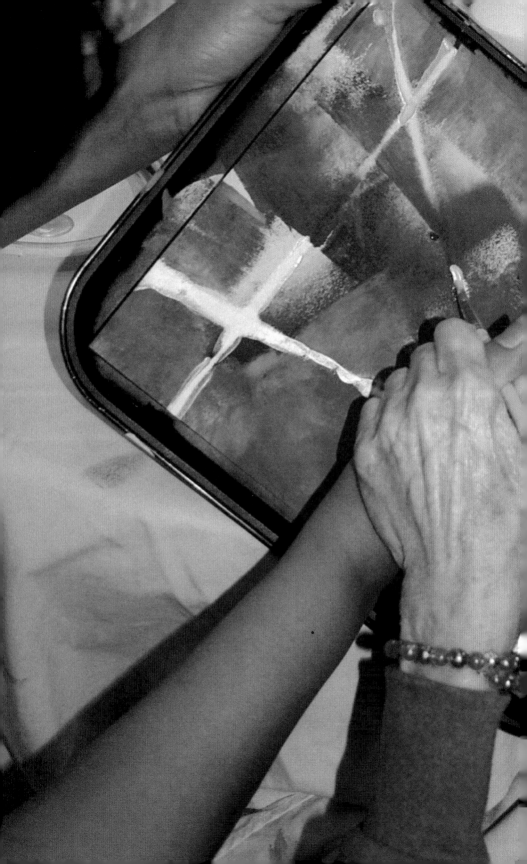

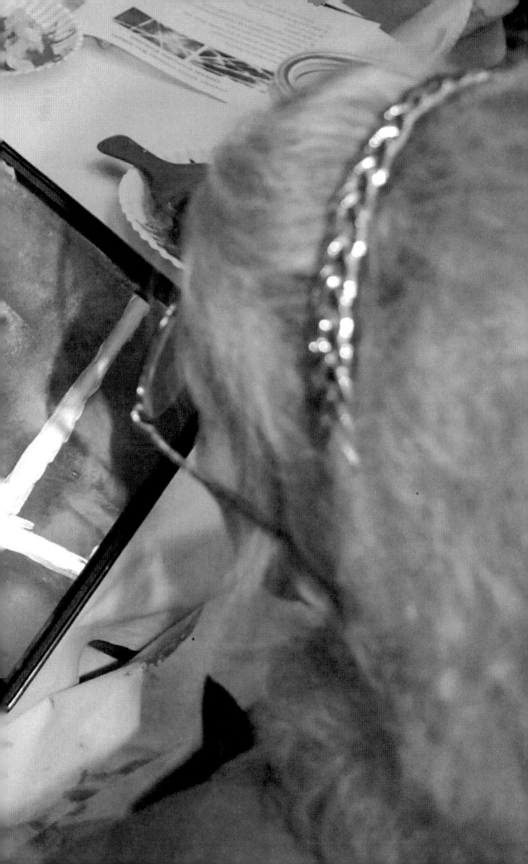

# Hand-Under-Hand Technique

This guiding and assisting technique provides a care partner with an amazing connection. It is a helping technique that provides both connection between them and protection for both parties. It promotes a physical touch connection that is friendly, comforting, and attention-getting without being intrusive or over-bearing. It also provides a system of feedback and communication between the person living with dementia and the person who is trying to interact or provide support and help. Hand-under-hand uses the much practiced and automatic connection between the eye and hand to form a closed circuit between the person who is struggling to understand words and tasks and objects and the care partner who knows what should be done, but can't find the phrase or gesture that allows that individual to process and do what is needed or wanted. It also provides a comforting and calming human connection using a familiar grasp and proprioception (deep pressure) in the palm at the base of the thumb. This eye-hand connection is one of the very first sensory-motor loops established in infants and is used almost endlessly throughout our daily lives. By using the palmar surface of the hand, and taking the person through the desired motion or movement, we are communicating with touch and movement, without the need for words. The use of hand-under-hand is multi-faceted:

1. It is used when greeting someone to sustain a physical connection, allowing the person to be more

comfortable with your presence in their intimate space. Having a comfortable hand hold makes it okay to be close to you. It is very different than a normal handshake that can be uncomfortable to sustain and which feels awkward after a few seconds. By having a hand-under-hand grasp, you will be able to tell if the person is enjoying your presence or wants you to allow them more space or less interaction without having to be come distressed or upset. If they keep trying to let go of you, let go and move back a little further. They may need a break or may not want you in their intimate space (within arm's reach) at that moment.

2. It can be used when helping someone move around. It provides greater stability and support as well as a feedback loop. Since the arm is the rudder that guides the ship, by rotating the forearm outward or inward

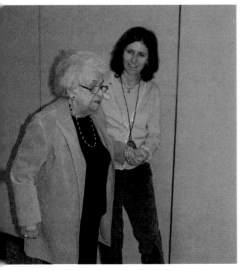

*Guiding Mobility*

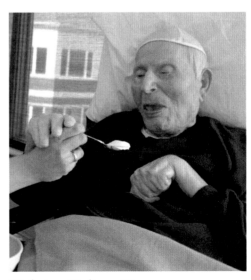

*Helping Deliver Care*

we can direct the walking path. By tipping the forearm down we can indicate physically the cue to sit down in a seat or on the commode, or on the bed. By tipping the forearm upward we can help the person stand upright. When used in combination with a gesture of pointing it can help provide direction and reassurance when moving through the environment in the later stages or when in an unfamiliar setting or on uneven surfaces. Because the care partner is close to the person, the awareness of balance, coordination, fear, or distress is telegraphed and can be responded to in a timely manner.

3. Hand-under-hand is essential during the Amber, Ruby, and Pearl Gem stages. It provides the care partner with a way to help the person understand the action being requested and can use the care partner's dexterity to operate the tool or utensil while the person living with dementia is still actively participating and moving their body parts toward their body (hand to mouth, hand to chest), as they have done for their entire lives. This automatic loop allows people living with dementia a sense of both control and involvement. It provides the helper with a way to get feedback on preferences, understanding, readiness and willingness to participate. It provides a way to do with, not do to or do for.

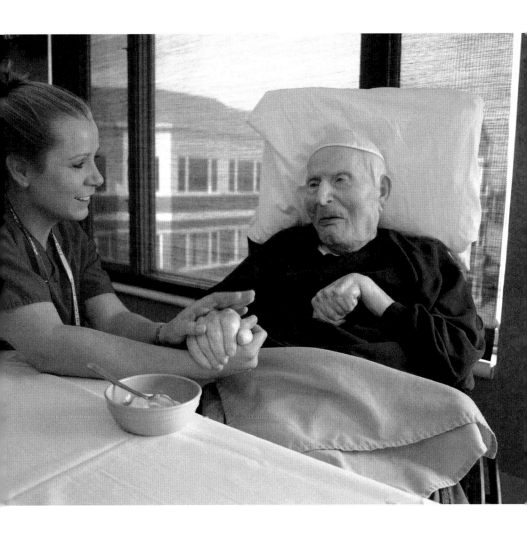

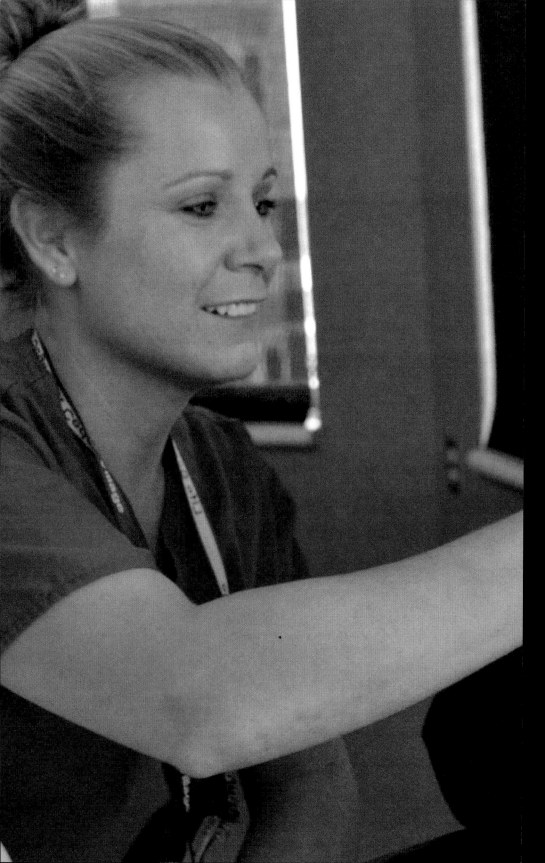

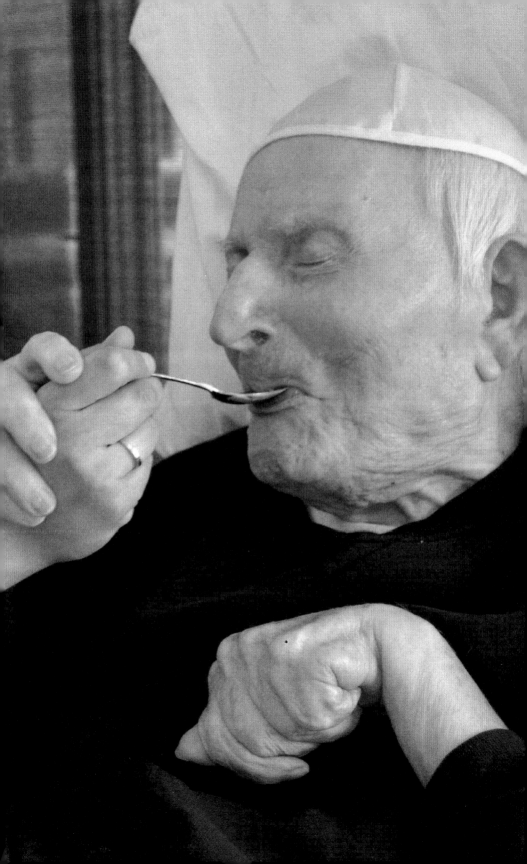

# How to Greet and Connect

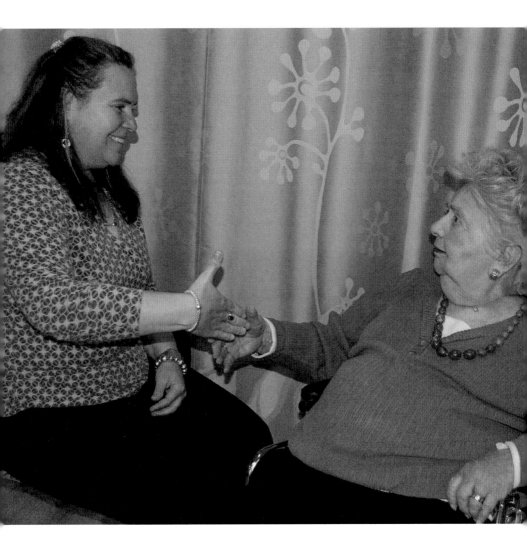

1. | Offer hand in a typical handshake.

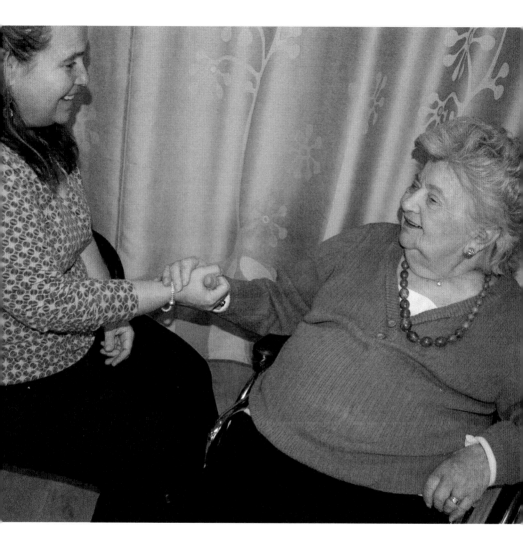

**2.** Shift your hand hold to having your thumbs locked, and fingers along the base of each other's thumbs.

# Comforting and Connecting

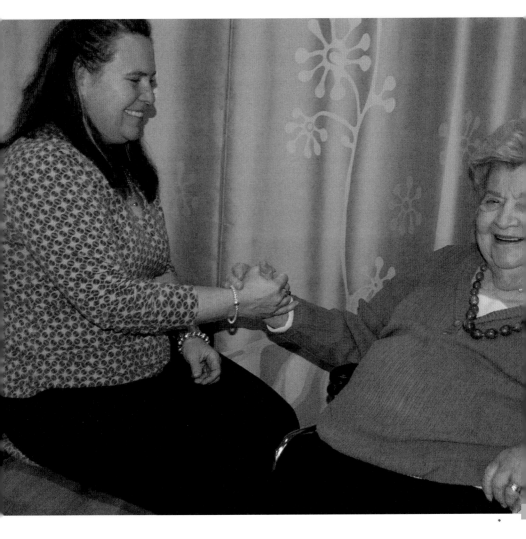

**3.** Then move into hand-under-hand position for comfort–your hand is *under* the person you are helping.

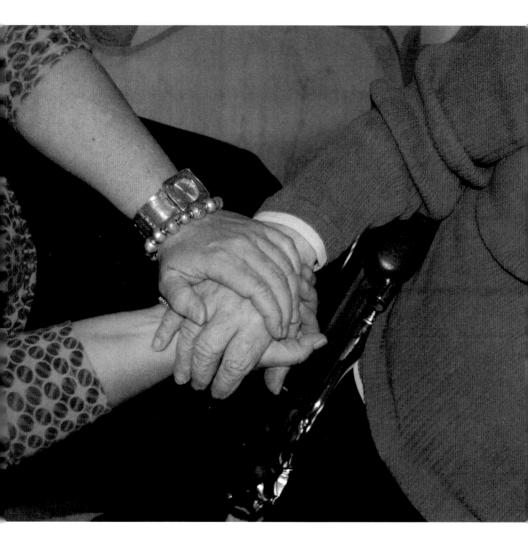

**4.** Lay your other hand over, to make a "comfort" sandwich–encourage eye contact and attention in a friendly way.

# A Positive Physical Approach for Someone with Dementia (PPA)

1. Knock on door or table to get attention and signal your approach.

2. Stop moving at the boundary between public and personal space–6 feet out–get permission to enter or approach.

3. Open hand motion near face and smile–look friendly and give the person a visual cue–make eye contact– open hand near face–cues eyes to look there.

4. Call the person by preferred name *or* at least say "Hi!"– avoid endearments.

5. Move your hand out from near your face to a greeting handshake position–make sure they notice your hand out to shake–then stand tall and move forward *slowly*.

6. Approach the person from the front–come in within 45 degrees of center-visual.

7. Move slowly–one step/second, stand tall, don't crouch down or lean in as you move toward the person.

8. Move toward the right side of the person and offer your hand–give the person time to look at your hand and reach for it, if s/he is doing something else–offer, don't force.

9. Stand to the side of the person at arm's length–respect intimate space and be supportive not confrontational– but don't go too far back–stay to the front-visual.

10. Shake hands with the person–make eye contact while shaking.

11. Slide your hand from a shake position to hand-under-hand position–for safety, connection, and function.

12. Give your name and greet–"I'm (name). It's good to see you!"

13. Get to the person's level to talk–sit, squat, or kneel if the person is seated and stand beside the person if s/he is standing.

14. *Now,* deliver your message…

# Approaching When the Person is Distressed

1. Look concerned, not too happy, if the person is upset.

2. Let the person move toward you, keeping your body turned to the side (supportive–not confrontational).

3. If the person is seated and you *don't* get permission to enter personal space–turn sideways and kneel at six feet out–offer greeting and handshake again–look for an okay to come into their personal space–it will usually come at this time (submissive posture).

4. After greeting…try one of two options…
   a. "Sounds like you are (give an emotion or feeling that seems to be true)…"
   b. Repeat the person's words to you…If s/he said, "Where's my mom?" you would say, "You're looking for your mom (*pause*)…tell me about your mom…" If the person said "I want to go home!", you would say, "You want to go home (*pause*)…Tell me…about your home…"

# Basic Cues with Dementia

- Knock and announce self.
- Pause at six feet.
- Greet and smile.
- Move slowly with hand offered in handshake position.
- Move from the front to the side.
- Greet with a handshake and your name.
- Slide into hand-under-hand hold.
- Get to the person's level.
- Be friendly–make a nice comment or smile.
- Give your message… simple, short, friendly.

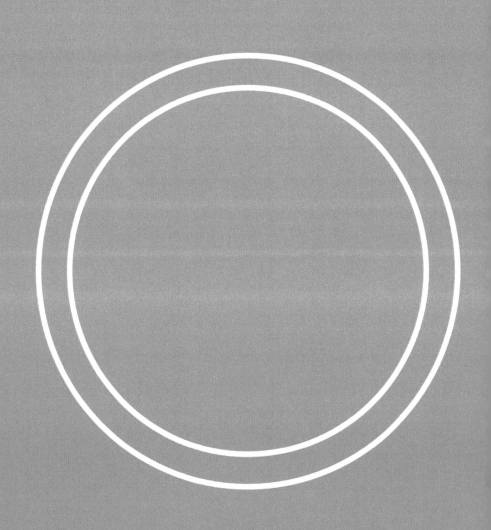

# Amber

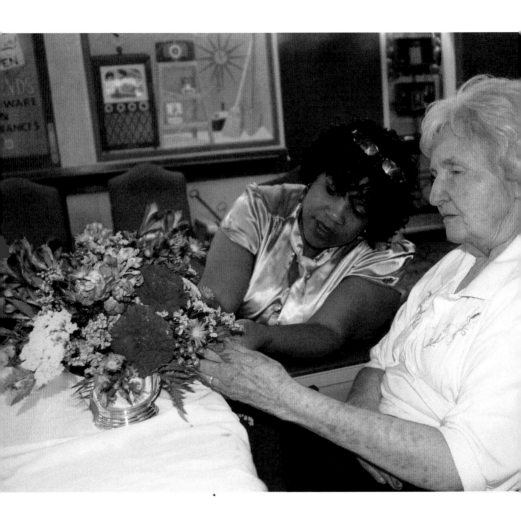

# Amber

## Yellow/Gold, Caution Light, Caught in a Moment of Time

### *Middle Stages*

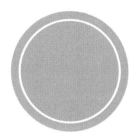

I am not rigid or hard anymore. I am softer and more malleable when you look at the whole day, but when I am caught in a moment and focused on sensation or the experience, I am stuck. You will need to wait and try again in a short while. If you are trying to get me to do something or get care completed, you will need to stop and give me a break, or I might become verbally or physically distressed.

I have limited safety awareness and don't understand much of the *why* behind what you do and are trying to get me to do or not do. I want what I want and like. What I don't like or can't tolerate, I won't do. I am *not* always aware of tasks and how things relate to one another.

I have no ability to delay or wait. You will need to respond to me ASAP for safety and opportunities to engage!

Although I may not know who you are to me (relationship), I will frequently know whether I like you and want to be with you or not, mostly based on how you look, sound, move, smell, and respond.

I may seem very ego-centric/self-focused. I am, not because I want to be, but because my brain is really seeking out sensations it likes and working to avoid what it doesn't like. I am not aware that I get too close, take your things, damage things, act child-like, or hurt your feelings or sensibilities, but I still want to have fun, enjoy myself, get connected, do my own thing, meet my needs. I am less aware of your needs and expectations.

I am also seeing objects and items, but not always remembering what they are or how to use them. Sometimes I can, sometimes I can't. This means you will need to secure spaces and items that could harm me, as I might try to handle them or use them without guidance or understanding (razor, sharp knife, deodorant, insurance papers, heirlooms, temperature controls, exit access). This also means I may not understand food as food, *but* you should also provide me with plenty of things I can interact with and use and enjoy.

Using my eye-hand skill is really important. It will help me maintain my dexterity skills as long as possible and allow me to practice and use brain circuitry that connects sensation and motor control. The value of what I am doing is in the *doing*, not in the product. I want and need to do things over and over at times. These experiences should be based on what I am enjoying and engaging with, not on what I have done before. Simple sorting or manipulative tasks may seem too easy, but I like easy, it makes me feel skilled and competent.

Because my behaviors are not usually typical for me when I was at my prime and are often based on my sensory preferences of the *moment*, it may be really hard for you to spend much time with me. It may surprise you when I investigate, touch, take, handle, smell, taste, take apart, or otherwise engage with items, people, or animals the way I do. It is a function of how my brain is processing incoming data and providing me with input.

I may not be able to tolerate some personal care routines that I once thought were essential to me. It is largely based on how my brain is handling sensory data. Typically, four areas of my body become *more* sensitive while others provide much less information. The lips/tongue/mouth area, the palms of the hands and fingertips, the soles of the feet and toes, and genitalia are sensory rich areas. As I lose more wiring and storage in my brain, I still feel these areas, so any care activities that involve these areas may distress me, now that I am an Amber. This may include: taking pills; shaving or facial hair removal, mouth care and dentures, eating and drinking (temperatures, tastes, and textures); hand washing and nail care; foot washing; shoes; toenail care, and going to the restroom, wiping, and changing briefs. It typically helps to pick up on my state, and back off if it isn't working, then re-approach in just a few minutes— possibly adjusting something to better match how I am right then.

Although I am hypersensitive in selected areas, I am not as aware of other parts of my body, this means I do not always feel what is wrong or pick up on my body's cues. I will typically become incontinent, may not recognize the importance of eating or drinking, do not know that I have had an accident, can't tell you that I am hurting, tired, hungry, thirsty, need to use the bathroom, am cold or too hot, or have something stuck in my teeth or shoe. I may over-react to something simple or under-react to something major. My wiring is fraying and dissolving.

## *Helpful Tips for Ambers* |

1. Use my behaviors to guide your responses! Be prepared for my sensory needs and tolerance issues. Plan to keep visits short, if it is hard to be with me. Better five *good* minutes than an hour of distress.

2. Look. Listen. Feel. Smell. Taste. Try hard to figure out the sensations I am seeking, avoiding, wanting, disliking *and* then try to either help me get what I want or reduce what is bothering me. It is better to *think* twice and act once, rather than being too quick and then having to try again and again.

3. Sometimes the best thing to do is take a *time-out*. Step away for a few minutes, breathe deeply and completely, then try to re-approach and re-connect using visual-verbal-touch cues that seem to match up with what I am doing at the moment.

4. Be willing to *slow down* or *speed up* to match me first, *then* gradually change the rhythm and pattern to reach a more comfortable level, without trying to get me to *stop*

or *get going* by opposing or blocking me.

5. Help the team come up with a list of sensory experiences and preferences based on what you have noticed and observed as well as getting input from others at different times and locations.

6. If you know any, share my past preferences related to:

   a. What I liked to look at and explore visually– any types of pictures, videos, or sight-based items I seemed to really connect with.
   b. What I liked to hear–musical and auditory preferences, volume preferences, any accent or speech factors that seem to make a difference.
   c. What touch and movement sensations I like and what I seem to avoid: being touched versus touching, types of textures and temperatures (for food and drink as well as handling) space from others, speed of movement, any rhythmic actions or movements (dancing, walking, exercising, rocking, swaying).
   d. Olfactory stimulation (smells) that calms or stimulates as well as smells to avoid or that I have disliked or have sensitivity to from past life experiences.
   e. Taste preferences and favorite flavors or recipes or food or drink. Items I have disliked.

7.  It will be important to *simplify* my world, tasks, expectations, and interactions–*not* infantilize, just simplify.

8.  When greeting me and offering me cues, exaggerate visual responses, use more automatic social greetings and movement encouragement, limit verbal information and instructions, and use hand under hand guidance and assistance when attempting to help me rather than doing things to me or for me.

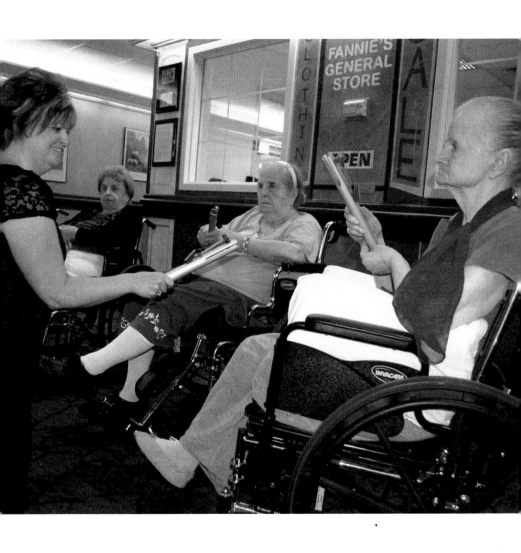

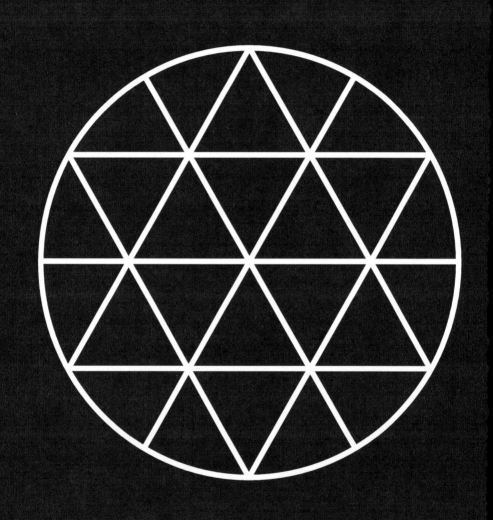

# Ruby

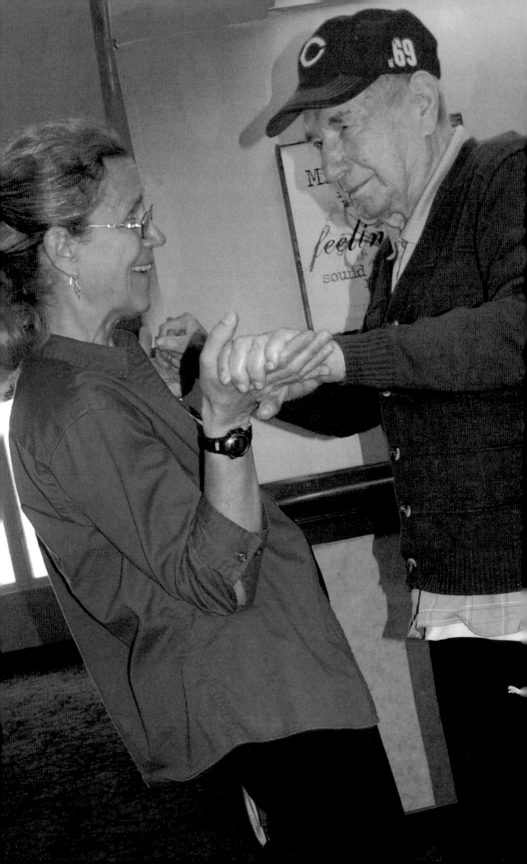

# Ruby

## Red, Stop Light, Hidden Depths

### Late Stage Changes

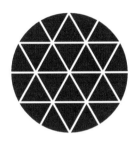

My brain is still trying to work, but it is struggling to understand the world around me. I still have deep, rich moments, but they are fewer and harder to see from your perspective. My fine details skills and abilities are failing, but my big movements and automatic actions, words, and reactions are frequently still present. There is a red light for changing gears or changing what I am doing. I am more likely to repeat what I am doing than switch to doing something new, unless I get clear, strong, multi-modal cues that help me make the shift. I am slowing down in all areas of ability, so if you try to get me to go too fast I am likely to shut down, resist, try to get away from you, or become frightened and immobilized latching on to where I am for dear life.

I still have some automatic speech, some rhythm to my speech, pick up your rhythms in speech, and can generally still sing or hum along and sometimes dance much better than I walk. If it happens automatically, I can do it better. But I do get stuck.

1.  I am losing fine motor in my eye function, but keeping big vision skills. My vision is changing. I am becoming monocular. My brain can no longer take the data coming in through each eye and superimpose the images so that I can see in 3-D. The options are double vision or ignore one image so the other is clear. Typically I will have no depth perception, although I will still see things. I misjudge distances. I may think a support is closer than it is, that a pattern in the carpet is something to be picked up, that a change in flooring is a step, or that a doorway is a hole or too small to get through. I am also not aware that there is a bigger world other than what I see. This means I can get stuck in corners, behind doors, in a room and not know how to get out. I can also trip over large objects and anything in my path that I don't notice when I am moving toward something I want or like. When I don't see something I will not know it exists, so when I turn around to sit down, I may not realize there is a chair there and keep walking looking for a place to sit.

2.  I am losing fine motor in my hands and fingers. I tend to hold, take, carry, wipe, grasp, and pinch with my thumb rather than use my fingers and manipulate items. I do not have good judgment on my grip strength and if I am not looking at something may forget I have it in

my hand.

3. I am losing fine motor in my feet and toes, but I am keeping my big movements and either a desire to move or I may develop an intense fear of falling. This leads to a continued desire for movement, but lack of balance and coordination when doing it or increasing immobility due to my fear of falling, because I know I am unstable. I am able to do automatic movements and actions, but if I think about it or have to plan it out, I have more difficulty. I get stuck easily when I can't figure out what to do or how to do it. Pulling or pushing me is very scary and it feels like you are trying to make me fall or hurt me. I am losing the ability to use utensils and tools, and do bilateral fine motor tasks such as buttoning, zipping, spearing with a fork, using a toothbrush on my own, etc.

4. I am losing fine motor in my lips, tongue, and mouth. I can suck and swallow either a bite or a drink, but if it is mixed I may choke (soup with chunks in the liquid, big bites with drinks). I may also "pocket food" in my cheek, as I am less aware of the sides of my mouth and can't control the muscles as well. I may also suck on items that are hard to manage and spit them back out or hold them in my mouth not being sure what to do with it.

In addition to the loss of fine motor skills, I am less aware of my body and the incoming sensory information from most of my body and organ systems but there are some locations that are hot spots for sensation. I feel strongly in these areas and may over-react when you do anything to me, if I don't understand or get it. These areas are my lips, tongue and mouth (especially right in the front), my fingers and finger nails, the soles of me feet and toes, and genitalia.

I am generally less interested in eating meals. I may graze more than sit down and eat a whole meal.

I tend to lose weight as I become more Ruby-like. I may be burning calories faster or having more trouble eating. Watch for signs and signals of hunger or thirst in my behavior, I generally won't be able to tell you, I don't know what I am feeling.

I may get injured and not seem to be aware of it. I may be in pain, but since I have limited body awareness, I don't know where or what is bothering me, so I might just seem more irritated or agitated.

Everything is slowing down and I can only handle limited stimulation at a time. I take much more time to process, so I need you to slow down and break things down more.

## Helpful Tips for Rubies

1. Slow down–it takes me longer to figure things out, do things, process anything, react.

2. Use the automatic when possible–I get rhythm, music, greetings, movements, not the details or specifics that I have to initiate, select, or sequence.

3. Break tasks down into small steps. You need to think it through, before you get started. First, determine where you want to end up, but remember to present only one step at a time for me.

4. Work on demonstrating and showing me what you want me to do, rather than telling or getting louder.

5. Start where I am, and then gradually shift gears until you help me get to the new state of motion or activity desired.

6. Plan the day out to have a balance of restful and active periods and plan to help me transition slowly and gradually from one to the other.

7. Plan to manage the sensory and physical environment for calming or stimulating cues depending on what I need at that time.

8. Use hand-under-hand-guidance for movement and pointing with your other hand for direction indication in order to let me know where to go or what you want me to notice.

9. Guide and cue, don't push or pull or force. The more you "push it," the more I will react and push back or resist.

10. Use hand under hand to provide and touch or care as it gives me more information that makes sense to my brain and limits the sense of sensitivity in key care areas.

11. Use your voice to engage and encourage, but limit talking, especially if I am trying to move away from you, the noisy area, or crowded space or activity. Be willing to be silent with me.

12. Use what is calming to me, all senses, to help me settle and what is stimulating to help me get going again.

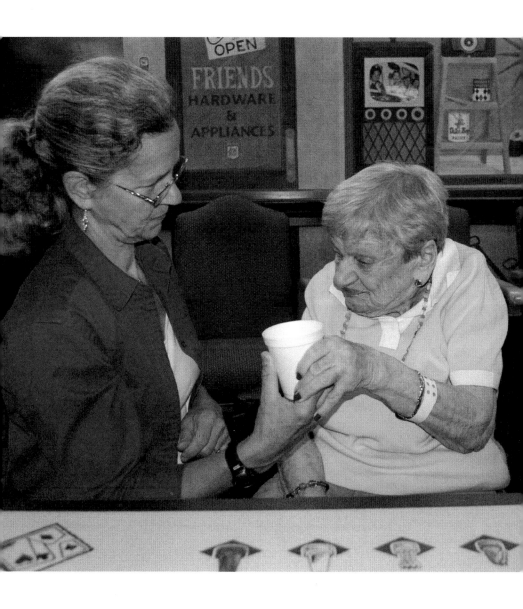

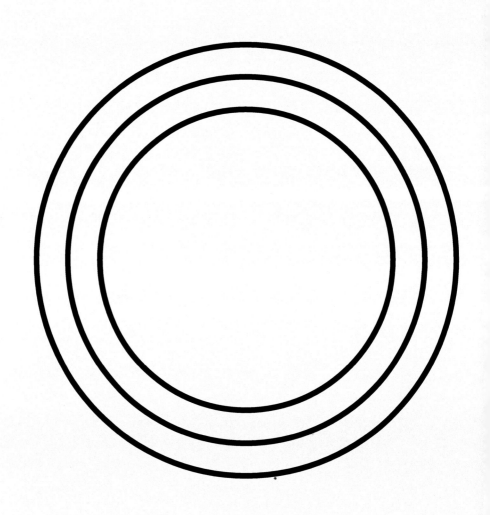

# Pearl

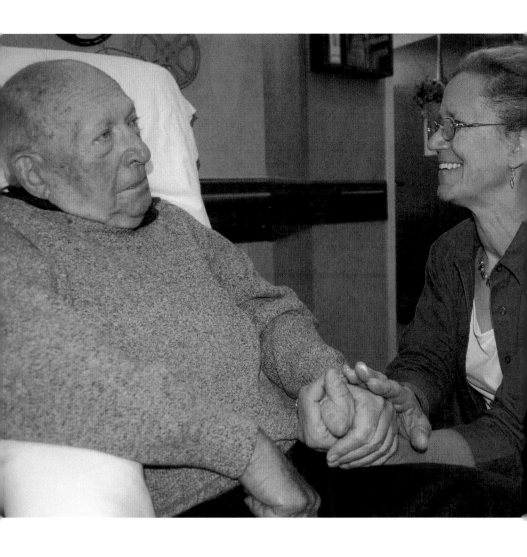

# Pearl

## In a Shell, Layer Upon Layer, Quiet Beauty

### *Late Changes, End of the Journey*

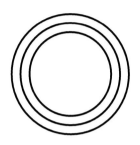

My brain is losing its ability to guide and direct my body. The control system for movement, interacting, responding, processing, and responding is failing. I am still here, but I am getting ready to leave.

Just like an oyster in a shell, I am hidden inside the shell of my body. Much of what my body does is ruled by reflexes. My muscles tend to be active and turned on most of the time. So I do tend to have contractures–they can't be fixed.

I startle easily and tighten up even more with quick movements, loud sounds, changes in light, unexpected touch, etc.

I spend much of time, resting or seeming unaware of much of the world around me, but there will be moments when I become alert and responsive–the shell opens and you can see me shine through–the pearl.

I am struggling to understand what you say, if you only use words and you get loud I may shut down and retreat.

I tend to respond best to familiar voices and rhythms and touches and gradual and gentle movements.

It takes a while for me to open up, but I may shut down in an instant and fade away. My balance is very poor. I may not be aware of leaning or sitting in one position for a long time.

Letting me know you are there, and that you are going to help me move, and then gradually shifting me is much better than thinking that because I am not awake and alert, it is better to just hurry and get it over with.

Helping me eat is a slow process and it is hard when I don't want more and yet you recognize that if I don't take in more food or drink, I will become dehydrated or malnourished.

I am not very interested in food or drink and I am starting to have trouble with coordinating swallowing and breathing. If you try to get me to take in what I can't manage, I will aspirate (food or drink will go into my lungs rather than into my stomach). Even when I do take in these items, I may not be able to get them to go into the right place. Just because I am not coughing, it doesn't mean I am not having swallowing problems. Sometimes my brain can't recognize the problem, so it doesn't react. This means I may develop pneumonia and be unable to fight it.

It is important to remember that it is normal for me to have muscle wasting and weight loss, that I may develop wounds that don't heal because I do not have enough protein processing, that I am very prone to infections, because my brain doesn't recognize and organize a response to infections.

It is critical to get through your grieving to accept that my condition is a terminal condition. The things you are seeing are just the symptoms of the ending of the disease. All your efforts to try to hang onto me to fix the pieces, will not change the big picture, all systems are failing.

The gift is that my body and brain are preparing for this. As I eat less and less and drink less and less, my brain is able to release endorphins. This allows me to not be distressed or in pain. I will not be hungry or thirsty when this happens. If you are ready, you may be able to offer me the greatest gift of all, by letting me know it is alright to go. I may not be able to leave you easily without your permission, after all, I do still care inside this shell, in moments when I am able to process and respond.

## Helpful Tips for Pearls |

1. Take time to observe me and check out how and where I am before approaching.

2. Determine how alert and aware I am.

3. If I am away use your voice and touch in a friendly and rhythmic way to bring me back to alertness and awareness.

4. If I am present, use the moments to connect and interact with me, using multi-model cues of

sight, sound, touch, smell, and possibly tastes But go slow and give me time to take in information, process it, and then respond.

5. Use the time we are together to be with me, not just care for me.

6. Always keep one hand still on a shoulder, hip, hand, or back, when you are doing something with the other hand. That way I have a better sense of where you are and I don't lose you.

7. Consider *body* experiences to allow me to have time that I can enjoy–cuddling close, stroking a pet, feeling the sun or a breeze on my face, hearing deep chimes or a chant or favorite prayer or poem or reading. Use smells that I seem to enjoy, modeling sniffing deeply to help me know what to do.

8. Offer me sips and tastes, but be less concerned about getting me to eat or drink. It should be about what I like, not about what is good for me at this point.

9. Talk to me, and with me, as if I were sitting right there with you; I am. Please don't talk about me as though I am an object or in third person.

10. Create opportunities for me to engage and respond, but don't force it or expect it. *I am doing the best I can.*

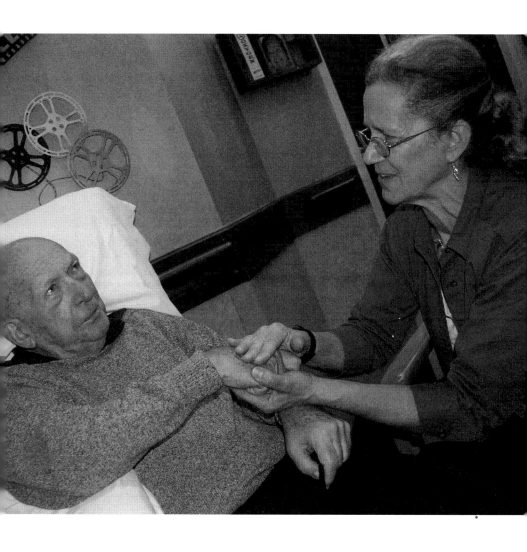

**Sapphire**

- Physical assist for hard-to-do tasks or personal care

- Will vary based on the physical and sensory issues facing the person

- If the condition is progressive, good idea to start talking about future options and what if…

- More well-designed visual, auditory, and just-right physical cues to support the person's abilities and compensate for missing pieces

**Diamond**

- Daily/weekly check-in on other health issues that are changing or are critical (new diagnosis, change in meds, new treatment)

- System to monitor finances, medications, transportation, pet or spouse care, and environmental safety

- Notification of events in a way that matches the person's need to know and ability to hold onto the information–a little in advance or just before

- Interactions that make the person feel special, valued, and engage me in ways I find acceptable

- May need a family meeting with a skilled facilitator to try to help everyone process what is happening and what should be done

| Gem | *Support Needed* |
|---|---|

**Emerald**

- Daily structure–more support and guidance may be needed in the afternoon and evening due to "wearing out" or increased distress about not being where and when the person thinks they are or should be

- Things that feel and look right to the person

- Balance of productive, self-care, leisure, and restorative programming each day–not able to do it without help

- Visual cues come first and then verbal information (not infantilized), making sure to match the visual to verbal–check in for comprehension

- Touching done with permission and friendly, not forced

- More than one care partner needed–for breaks, variety, and well-being of all

- Time to consider a secured or more closely monitored care location if and when the person physically tries to go to another time or place (best predictor of elopement/wandering is having done it before–others are illness, anything new or different is happening…, emotional distress, flight history)

**Amber**

- 24/7 monitoring for safety and engagement with physical guidance and assistance to complete care tasks, guide and direct, and stimulate interest or reduce distress

- An environment that is protective and yet provides positive stimulation and experiences

- Personnel and care partners who are alert to the person's needs and interests and respond quickly and effectively without being judgmental or parental

- Care partners who want to be with the person and are able to guide and redirect, stop and retry later, interpret nonverbal cues and behaviors, and know how to take time-outs when they need breaks rather than become frustrated with the person

- Programming that provides smooth transitions from stimulation to relaxation throughout the day and into the evening, possibly at night (if there is nighttime wakefulness)

- A team of care partners needed, so that everyone can get rest and be ready to help the person who is only able to be in the moment.

| Gem | *Support Needed* |
|---|---|

**Ruby**

- 24/7 physical assistance/supervision and programming to meet the increasing hands-on and physical care needs, and for those using their mobility skills, there will be times two care partners may be needed to help with movement and care

- Daily routines that are structured but flexible based on the person's rhythm of wake sleep and provide help in transitioning from active to quiet and quiet to active

- Spaces and supports that allow and encourage the just right amount of movemen and mobility but are protective and limited to create safer options as the person's fine motor skills are disappearing

- Sensory rich environments that use the person's background and preferences to create opportunities for sights, sounds, textures, temperatures, movements, smells, and tastes that appeal–stimulate or calm depending on what is needed

- Individualized engagement opportunities, but balanced and provided in places and spaces that create a sense of security, familiarity and acceptance.

| Gem | *Support Needed* |
|-----|------------------|

**Pearl**

- 24/7 monitoring for needs and care
- Physical care throughout 24 hours as needed and tolerated
- Responsive care that uses non-verbal cues to guide what is done and how it is done
- Specialized seating and sleeping options, based on postures and contractures
- Sensory rich environment that provides sensation that comforts and stimulates on an individualized routine

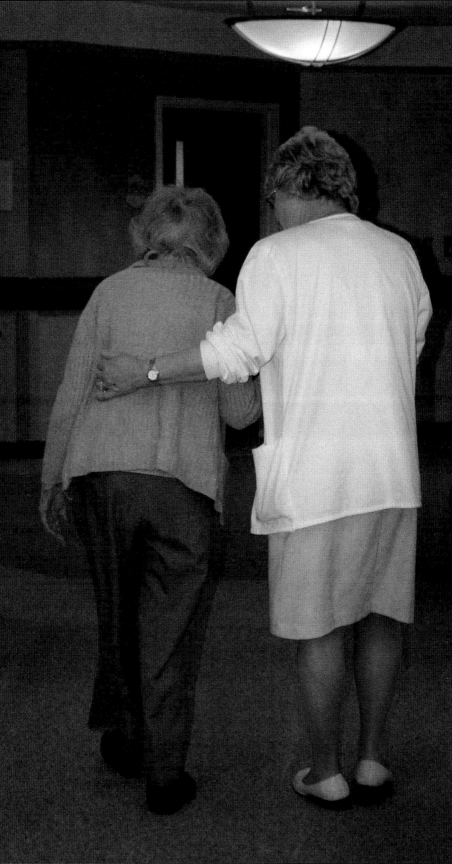

# Conclusion

When someone you care about develops dementia it will eventually change almost everything about that person. Dementia is not a memory problem, it is brain failure. As caregivers, we have choices. We can try to fight back and battle the disease. The problem with this strategy is that the disease is hidden inside the person we care about, and it often feels like we are angry and upset with them. We can give up and just let it happen, seeing only what we are losing and the shell that remains. Or we can choose to commit ourselves to learning how to let go of what is fading, but celebrating and using what remains at any point in time. We can choose to become care partners on this journey, not caregivers or those who step away because "she doesn't know who I am anymore." Each person must make the choice for themselves. You cannot make it for another.

If you choose to become a care partner, the journey will be hard. There may be times it hurts and times when you need a break or a partner yourself. You will make mistakes. You are human and you cannot get it right the first time, every time. When you are trying to think for another, it doesn't always work out the way we plan. The goal in dementia is to plan for the worst probabilities, but celebrate the best moments!

The one constant in this ever-changing condition can be your commitment to travel with someone as they make the journey. To do this you must plan to change as the condition changes the person's ability to understand the world, to process incoming information and data, to respond or react to what happens and how it happens, and to even live in this world.

The following points are important to keep in mind:

- Many times when we are surprised or frustrated by something–it is not the person, it is the disease.

- We can use what we see, hear, feel, and experience with the person to guide our behavior.

- Interacting with the person we knew will require us to work hard–not just do what comes naturally in many situations.

We must learn to respond, not react–there may be moments when the only thing we can do is stop, and step away to re-gather ourselves…first, do no harm.

To be successful care partners we will need to let go of what was, what should be, how the person should be, how we should be, and live in the moment we are given.

By seeing each person as a Gem of great value, precious and unique, I hope this booklet helps each of you on your journey through this challenge called dementia.

—*Teepa*

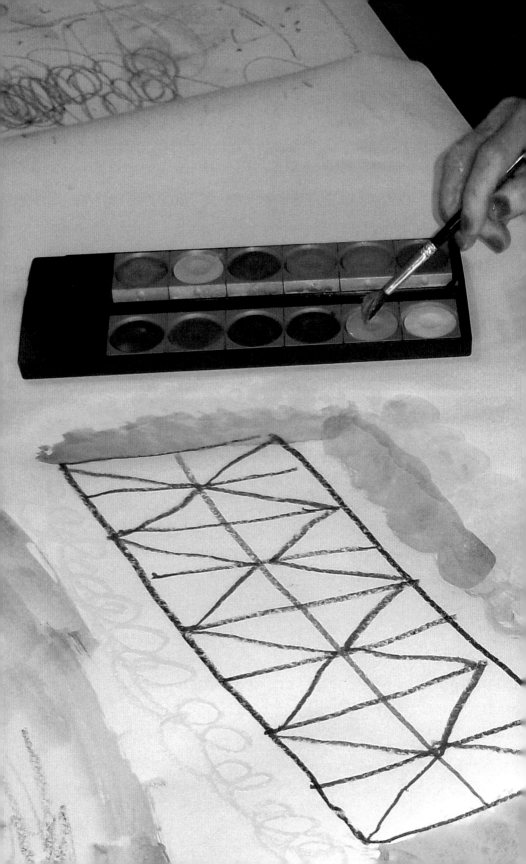

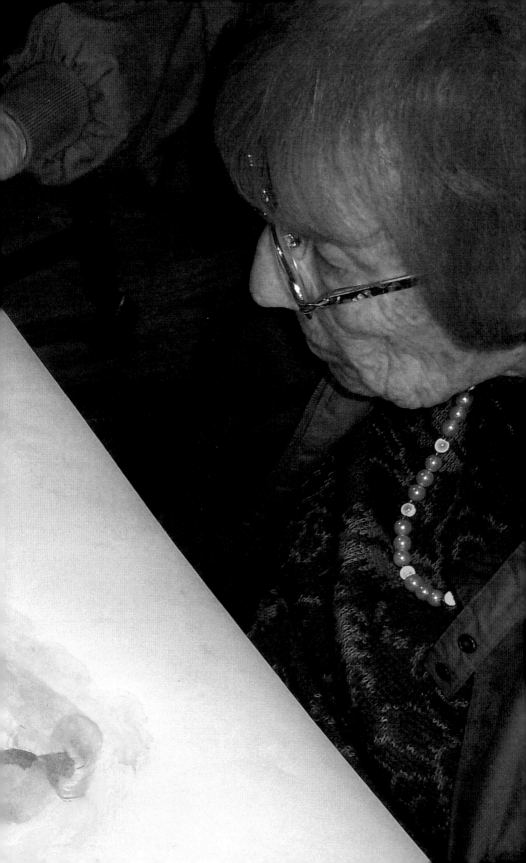

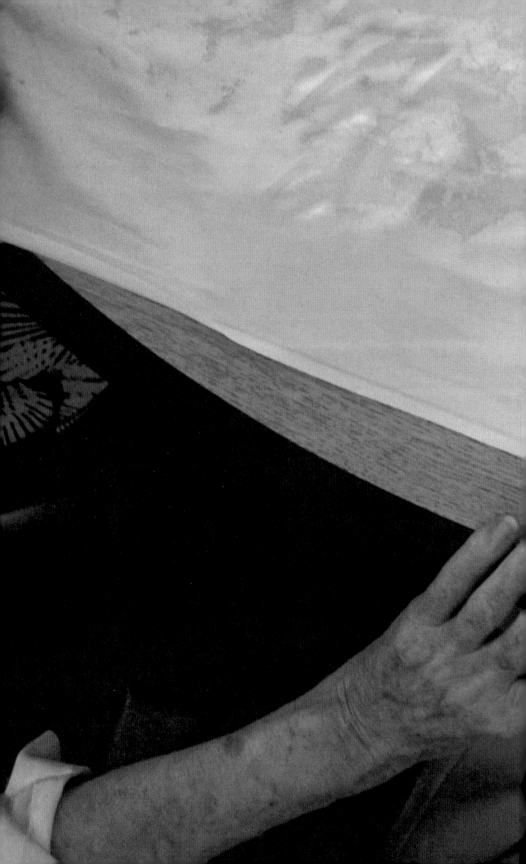

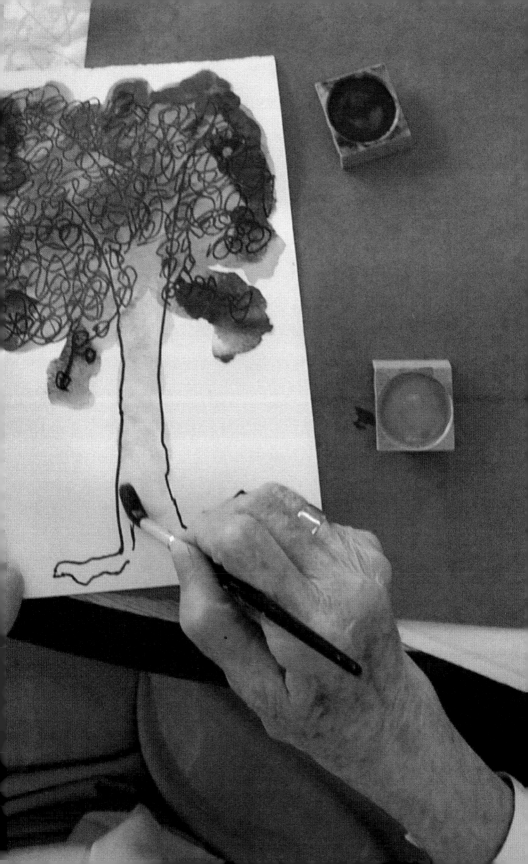

# Teepa's Background

Teepa Snow is a Master's prepared Occupational Therapist with over thirty years of clinical practice and teaching experience in a wide variety of educational and clinical settings. She has clinical appointments at Duke University School of Nursing, and the University of North Carolina at Chapel Hill School of Medicine. She has developed her knowledge and skills through her rich and diverse work and life experiences. She has worked in hospitals, rehabilitation centers, retirement communities, nursing homes, home care, hospice, and community settings. She has taught at universities and colleges from associate degree to post-doctoral level. She has worked closely with clinical researchers in geriatrics throughout her career and has extensive experience in neurological care settings, working with people who have had head injuries, strokes, and other central nervous system failures. She served as the lead trainer and educational director for the Alzheimer's Association in Eastern North Carolina, where she helped to develop training programs and videos that are used by national organizations to prepare caregivers for supporting someone with dementia.

She began her caregiving journey as a young girl when her grandfather came to live with the family and it became clear he was getting "senile." It turned out Teepa was much better at helping her grandfather get through the day than her mother, who became easily frustrated with repeated questions and unrealistic expectations. That early experience seemed to shape her career and direction. She later provided care and support to two other family members who developed forms of dementia.

These days, Teepa spends the majority of her time providing educational sessions for groups and associations across North America. She consults with selected organizations and agencies on program development, environmental design, and staff education and care provision. Such is her relationship with Cedar Village. Over the past five years, Cedar Village leaders and staff have implemented Dementia Care Specialist training throughout the community. With Teepa's support and guidance, together we are making a difference in the lives of people living with dementia and their families.

·

.

Made in the USA
Las Vegas, NV
24 October 2023